Menopause Reset

A Comprehensive Guide to Understanding
and Managing Menopause

Sally Davis

Table Of Contents

Introduction

This book is designed to provide you with a wealth of knowledge, practical advice, and support as you embark on this significant phase of your life.

Menopause is a natural biological process that marks the end of a woman's reproductive years. It is a transformative journey that brings about hormonal changes, physical adjustments, and emotional shifts. While every woman's experience is unique, there are common themes and challenges that many encounter during this time. This guide aims to shed light on these aspects and equip you with the tools to navigate this transition with confidence and grace.

In the pages that follow, we will delve into the various dimensions of menopause, exploring its physical, emotional, and psychological implications. We will address common symptoms such as hot flashes, night sweats, mood swings, and sleep disturbances, providing practical strategies for managing them effectively. Moreover, we will explore the impact of menopause on relationships, sexuality, and overall well-being, offering guidance to help you maintain a fulfilling and healthy lifestyle.

Throughout this guide, we will draw upon the latest research, medical expertise, and personal stories to provide you with a comprehensive understanding of menopause. You will find evidence-based information, empowering you to make informed decisions about your health and well-being. Additionally, we will discuss various treatment options, including hormone therapy, alternative therapies, lifestyle changes, and self-care practices, so that you can explore what works best for you.

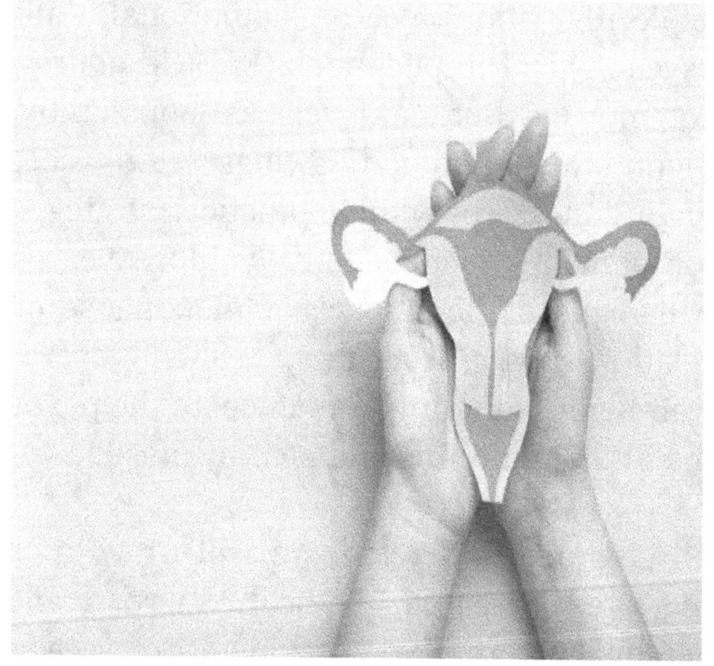

Menopause is not a time to fear or dread, but rather an opportunity for growth, self-discovery, and embracing the next chapter of your life. By arming yourself with knowledge and support, you can navigate menopause with confidence, reclaim your vitality, and embrace the possibilities that lie ahead.

Join us on this transformative journey, as we explore the complexities and joys of menopause, and empower you to thrive during this remarkable phase of womanhood.

Remember, you are not alone. Together, let's navigate menopause and celebrate the beauty and wisdom it brings.

Chapter 1 Basics

Menopause is the permanent cessation of menses for 12 months resulting from estrogen deficiency and is not associated with a pathology. The median age of menopause is 51. Most women experience vasomotor symptoms, but menopause affects many other areas of the body, such as urogenital, psychogenic, and cardiovascular. Patients are living longer, and women are spending up to one-third of their lives post-menopause.

Menopause is a routine, non-pathologic condition involving the permanent cessation of menses for at least 12 months. Menopause occurs in all menstruating females due to non-pathologic estrogen deficiency. The median age of menopause is 51. Most women experience vasomotor symptoms, but menopause can affect many areas, some of which are the urogenital and cardiovascular systems. This activity reviews the presentation, evaluation, and management of menopause and stresses the role of an interprofessional team approach to care for affected individuals.

As women grow older, their ovarian follicles diminish in number. There is a decline in granulosa cells of the ovary, which were the main producers of estradiol and inhibin. With the lack of inhibition from estrogen and inhibition of gonadotropins, follicle-stimulating hormone (FSH) and luteinizing hormone (LH) production increases. FSH levels are usually higher than LH levels because LH is cleared from the blood faster. The decline in estrogen levels disrupts the hypothalamic-pituitary-ovarian axis. As a result, a failure of endometrial development occurs, causing irregular menstrual cycles until they stop altogether.

Menopause may occur due to surgical procedures such as a hysterectomy with bilateral oophorectomy. Menopause can be caused by treatment for certain conditions, like endometriosis and breast cancer with antiestrogens and other cancers due to chemotherapy medications.

In the United States, approximately 1.3 million women become menopausal each year. It typically begins between the ages of 51 and 52. However, about 5% of women experience early menopause between the ages of 40 and 45. Additionally, 1% of women experience premature menopause before the age of 40 due to permanent ovarian failure that may be associated with sex chromosome abnormalities.

Menopause is a normal physiologic process in aging women in which the number of ovarian primary follicles quickly diminishes, such that there are inadequate amounts to respond to the effects of FSH. In turn, there is no LH surge, and ovulation does not take place, resulting in the decline of estrogen production and the cessation of menstruation. Moreover, LH and FSH go uninhibited and remain at high levels years after the onset of menopause. Small amounts of estrogen may still be produced via conversion from testosterone released by the adrenal glands, such that symptoms other than the discontinuation of periods may be negligible in some individuals.

Generally, no laboratory tests are required for the diagnosis of menopause. The diagnosis is clinically based on the patient's age, symptoms, and ruling out other conditions for patients older than 45 years old. Furthermore, symptoms may precede changes in laboratory values. However, an elevated serum FSH (greater than 40 mIU/mL) can be indicative of menopause (via ovarian failure), although it is insensitive. Additionally, drugs like estrogens, androgens, and hormonal contraceptives may alter lab results.

The United States Preventive Services Tasks Force suggests starting screening for osteoporosis at age 65 if normal risk factors are present. If osteoporosis is a concern (i.e., falls, fractures, medications), a dual-energy x-ray absorptiometry (DEXA) scan can be done. A T-score on DEXA of 1.0 to 2.5 is indicative of osteopenia, while a T-score greater than 2.5 is indicative of osteoporosis

Even though menopause is a physiological condition and not a disease, it has significant morbidity. Besides the increased risk of osteoporosis and fractures, the women also regain their risk for heart disease. In addition, the symptoms of menopause are poorly tolerated and lead to poor quality of life. The majority of these women are seen in clinical practice by the nurse practitioner, primary care provider, or internist.

Healthcare workers, including the nurse and pharmacist, should educate the patient on the physiology of menopause. Only those who are not able to tolerate the symptoms should be treated. It appears that many clinicians have started to use menopause as an opportunity to prescribe all sorts of treatments without solid evidence. If there is osteoporosis, a better option is the use of bisphosphonates. Hormonal agents should only be used for short periods and at the lowest dose to avoid complications.

The nurse should educate the patient on the increased risk of heart disease and emphasize prevention. A dietician should educate the patient about a healthy diet. The women should be encouraged to exercise regularly, discontinue smoking and maintain a healthy weight. Since menopause can also result in mood changes, a mental health nurse should offer counsel. Clinicians should ensure that women undergo a bone scan and eat a diet rich in calcium and vitamin D. The pharmacist should urge women not to take untested products and seek guidance from clinicians. Only with an interprofessional team approach can the morbidity of menopause be lowered.

Understanding the clock

The menopausal transition stage is where perimenopause primarily occurs. Earlier on in this stage, the menstrual cycle undergoes variability in its duration, such that the length of time between menstruations differs by 7 or more days each cycle. As this stage progresses, women typically experience amenorrhea for a period of 60 or more days. Once this occurs, women are in the late menopausal transition, which takes place for 1 to 3 years. Supportive lab work may show a variable elevated FSH level earlier on in the menopausal transition stage and an elevated FSH greater than 25 IU/L later on. The FSH greater than 25 IU/L is due to the decline of estrogen. At this stage, women may likely experience vasomotor symptoms.

Although the average age of menopause is 51, menopause can actually happen any time from the 30s to the mid-50s or later. Women who smoke and are underweight tend to have an earlier menopause, while women who are overweight often have a later menopause. Generally, a woman tends to have menopause at about the same age as her mother did.

Menopause can also happen for reasons other than natural reasons. These include:

Premature menopause. Premature menopause may happen when there is ovarian failure before the age of 40. It may be associated with smoking, radiation exposure, chemotherapeutic drugs, or surgery that impairs the ovarian blood supply. Premature ovarian failure is also called primary ovarian insufficiency.

Surgical menopause. Surgical menopause may follow the removal of one or both ovaries, or radiation of the pelvis, including the ovaries, in premenopausal women. This results in an abrupt menopause. These women often have more severe menopausal symptoms than if they were to have menopause naturally.

Perimenopause

Let's have a look at the three stages of the menopause itself. So we've got the perimenopause. This is the phase leading up to the menopause. This can last about three to five years, it just depends on you as an individual, how this is going to sort of pan out. You can start to feel your hormones changing a number of years before your periods actually start to change. So you can be getting completely normal, regular periods, everything just the exact same, and then you suddenly feel as if you're starting to get some menopause symptoms. You could end up with things like your hot flushes, joint aches, digestive problems, headaches, and stress palpitations as well. And these tend to be some of the common ones that would happen at this particular point.

The problem with these symptoms at this time is that they are not often associated with the menopause. So women, they'll start to get the stress palpitations and really worry about this or they start to get joint aches or digestive problems, and they will go along to the doctor and get tested, and the thing is, the tests will come back completely clear. And that's quite a worry because you know that something's not right, you know something's going on, but very often the doctor will say, "Well, there's nothing wrong with you. You just take painkillers or antacid tablets or something like that." So there's a lot of symptoms at this particular point that are often not realized that they are part and parcel of the menopause. If you are in the perimenopause, it's a good idea to just look at your general health at this particular moment in time and, if there is anything going on, maybe have a look and see whether it can be more associated with the menopause rather than anything else at all.

Now, in the perimenopause, at some point, you will find your periods starting to change. The menopause or the perimenopause, it's not a static state. Your hormones just don't fall gracefully and that's it. They can go up and down like a yo-yo, and you might find that for six months, you get one set of symptoms and then they disappear, and then you get another set of symptoms. So, during this phase of three to five years, you can actually end up getting a range of different menopause symptoms at different times. You know, if you start off getting hot flushes, that does not mean that you're going to get hot flashes, you know, every single day for the next five years. It doesn't actually work in that way.

Now, for some women, they may find that their periods start to get closer together, they might start to get a little bit heavier, they might start to get a little bit more prolonged. That normally means, at that point, that your progesterone is forming just that bit quicker than your estrogen. So these are sort of high estrogen symptoms.

Some women find that their periods start to tail off, they start to get further apart, they get lighter, they start to go missing. You might find you get one period and then miss them for four months, and then get another period, and so on. And this is normally an indication that your estrogen is falling that little bit quicker than your progesterone is falling.

But you can get a combination of both. You can get heavy periods for a year and then they suddenly start to tail off. And then at some point, you will find your periods just stop for good. Now, there are some lucky women that don't get any sign or any symptoms, their periods just stop and that's it. That's the menopausal stage. So, sometimes that does actually happen.

The menopause

So the next phase, once you think to yourself, "Oh, my periods have actually stopped." The menopause itself, believe it or not, is just the moment in time when your periods just stop for good. Problem is, you don't know your periods have stopped for good, until you've not had one for about two years. Now, there are some schools of thought that say you've gone through the menopause when you haven't had any periods for a year, but we actually find that quite a large number of women can go for a year or more without a period and then get one or two back again. Sometimes, you know, it's a last fling of their hormones. So, we tend to say, once you have not had any periods for two years, that you're through the menopause.

Now, this phase, from when your periods have stopped for good until the two years to stop, your hormones are still changing, so you can still get a number of symptoms at this particular point. And some women find that this is when they start to maybe get a little bit worse purely, because your hormones are falling that little bit further. However, the majority of women find that, as you approach the end of the two years, that the body has learnt to rebalance itself and that your symptoms will start to ease off. Now, the only problem here is that the length of time it takes for your symptoms to ease off can be very often linked to your general health; your lifestyle, stress management, and your diet. So this phase is very important where you still need to keep looking after yourself well.

Post-menopause

Now, once you've got to the two years without a period, you're then considered postmenopausal. And that's the point where your hormones will start to level off. It doesn't get to the point where you have no hormones at all, or that's very, very rare. Your body will learn to cope with a lower level of hormones.

That's the point when you can actually start to feel better. You can start to get your old self back, your body can cope, your energy will come back, and there's no reason at this point postmenopausal, when you can't actually feel as good, if not better than you did before. This is because you've got no hormonal ups and downs, there's far less emotional ups and downs going on as well.

So, this phase, the post-menopausal phase, can actually be a really great one. But again, you still need to keep looking after yourself well.

Remember everybody's menopause is unique

So, it's quite a complex situation and you must remember that every single one of you is going to have a completely unique menopause. And the information that I gave today is just a general guide. Some women will have really, really long menopauses, other women will have very, very short ones. And the combination of symptoms that you get at any given time, are going to be different to everybody else's.

Chapter 2 Menopause symptoms and what to do

Your relationships, social life, family life, career, and other aspects of your everyday life can all be significantly impacted by menopause and perimenopause symptoms.

Everyone will experience it differently. You can exhibit several symptoms or none at all.

Typically, symptoms appear months or even years before your periods cease. The term for this is the perimenopause.

HOT FLASHES

A drop in estrogen levels causes hot flashes. Your glands react to this by releasing more of other hormones, which change the thermostat in your brain and cause changes in body temperature. For many women, hormone treatment has been demonstrated to ease some of the discomfort associated with hot flashes. However, you and your healthcare practitioner shouldn't decide to start using these hormones until after weighing the risks and benefits.

The National Heart, Lung, and Blood Institute of the National Institutes of Health started the Women's Health Initiative (WHI) in 1991 to study more about women's health, particularly hormone treatment. The estrogen plus progestin study of women with uteruses and the estrogen-alone study of women without uteruses were the two studies that made up the hormone trial. Both trials came to an early conclusion after finding that hormone treatment raised the risk for various medical conditions while doing nothing to protect against heart disease. Studies done afterward revealed that women who started estrogen-plus-progestin treatment more than ten years after menopause had a higher chance of developing heart disease.

The WHO advises women to adhere to FDA recommendations for hormone therapy (estrogen-alone or estrogen-plus-progestin). It indicates that using hormone treatment won't help you avoid heart disease.

These medicines are recognized as effective treatments for the alleviation of mild to severe hot flashes as well as the signs of vulvar and vaginal atrophy. Although hormone treatment may be useful for preventing postmenopausal osteoporosis, it should only be explored for women who cannot take anti-estrogen medications but are at considerable risk of osteoporosis. The FDA advises using hormone therapy at the lowest dosage for the shortest amount of time necessary to meet therapeutic objectives. Postmenopausal women who use or are thinking about utilizing hormone treatment should speak with their medical professionals about the potential advantages and hazards.

Following are some helpful tips for dealing with heat flashes:

Wear layers so you can shed them as soon as a heat flash begins.

Avoid spicy meals, alcohol, coffee, tea, and other hot beverages, as well as other foods and drinks that might trigger hot flashes.

When a hot flash begins, sip a glass of cool water or fruit juice.

Reduce your level of tension. Hot flushes may develop under stress.

When you go to bed at night, have an ice pack or a thermos of cold water nearby.

Use breathable clothes, lingerie, and bedding made of cotton.

To discover what might cause your hot flashes, keep a journal or record of your symptoms.

LOW SEX DRIVE

Numerous physiological, psychological, and social factors can contribute to decreased libido (or sex desire). A woman's sex drive is shaped by her emotional and physical health, as well as her life events, personal and religious views, socialization, and present relationships.

Menopause, in certain ways, affects both the physical and psychological aspects of sex desire. Because estrogen levels drop precipitously after menopause, there is less interest in sex. Reduced lubrication from dry vaginal tissues brought on by lower estrogen levels may cause discomfort or even agony during sex, which may in turn impair sexual desire. Reduced blood flow also has an impact on general arousal and vaginal lubrication. As a result, a woman might not enjoy having sex as much and can find it challenging to have orgasms.

Effects of Falling Estrogen Levels During Menopause on the Body
Hot flashes, nocturnal sweats, and vaginal dryness are physical side effects of declining estrogen levels that can reduce sexual urge and motivation throughout the menopausal transition. The age-related decline in testosterone, however unrelated to menopause, may lessen desire in middle-aged women since these hormone levels affect sex drive and sexual feelings in women.

However, because reduced sexual desire in women has not been linked to testosterone levels in research studies, the specific function of testosterone in desire is complicated. Additionally, compared to women who go through natural menopause, some women who experience abrupt menopause (induced by the removal of both ovaries or by chemotherapy), which causes an instantaneous decline in both estrogen and testosterone, have a higher loss of desire. Interestingly, some ladies in the same circumstance don't experience a decline in desire.

A woman's desire for sexual activity during menopause and later may be influenced by a variety of different variables, not the least of which is a lower estrogen level. These consist of:

issues with bladder control
disruptions in sleep
Moodiness or worry
Mood changes
Stress
Medications

Health issues
problems in a relationship with a partner
For the majority of women, night sweats and other symptoms that cause libido loss do ultimately go away. Women who lack the protective benefits of hormones like estrogen are more susceptible to heart disease, weight gain, and other health issues.

While many women still engage in and enjoy sexual activity throughout menopause, for some, it becomes more of a burden. Women who are menopausal or postmenopausal may realize that they are less amenable to being touched or stroked and that they are less quickly aroused. And while many women and their partners may still experience closeness without engaging in sexual activity, other couples find it difficult to adjust to these changes.

CHANGING PERIODS

Your regular bleeding pattern may vary throughout perimenopause and menopause, which is one of the most obvious signs. Although some women have more erratic periods, most of us are used to monthly bleeding.

You could start to notice any of the following changes as you move toward menopause:

You could start skipping periods.
They may lighten up.
You can feel exhausted and drained as a result of them being longer or heavier.
They could even increase in frequency.
You can have flooding, where the period comes out in a gush, or you might pass clots.
Some women may abruptly cease for no apparent reason.

It's important to keep in mind that many women take hormones for contraception, which might alter their menstrual cycles. For instance, many women who use the MirenaTM coil, the progesterone-only pill, the implant, or a contraceptive injection find that their bleeding patterns shift or stop altogether. Even during perimenopause, the combined oral contraceptive pill can maintain regular menstruation.

Therefore, you cannot use altering bleeding patterns to determine whether you are in perimenopause or have gone through menopause if you are on hormones.

Why do periods change?
The coordination of multiple hormones (chemical messengers) is necessary for a monthly bleed to occur regularly.

To maintain your hormones in a monthly cycle, your brain and ovaries interact. The endometrium, or lining of the womb, is affected by ovarian hormones (estrogen and progesterone), which thicken it each month in preparation for caring for a pregnancy. Then, if you are not pregnant, it sheds, which is period-like bleeding.

Your hormones may go out of whack during perimenopause, and your brain and ovaries may no longer be able to communicate with one another. You don't experience that typical thickening and loss of your uterine lining.

You can experience inconsistent bleeding or perhaps no bleeding at all. When estrogen levels are low during menopause, the lining of the womb stops thickening, and bleeding ceases.

Other causes of irregular bleeding include fibroids, endometrial polyps (polyps in the lining of the uterus), and, less frequently, precancerous and cancerous alterations. In addition to the vagina and vulva, the cervix can also cause bleeding, which is why it's critical to maintain a schedule for cervical smears.

Menopause-related hemorrhage

Vaginal bleeding after menopause, or bleeding after your periods have ceased for more than a year, is a problem for some women. The term for this is postmenopausal bleeding. Even spotting or bleeding that appears brown or pink or has only occurred once after menopause has to be examined by a doctor.

Postmenopausal bleeding is often caused by a benign condition, but it may sometimes be an indication of malignancy. If detected early, this kind of cancer is easily treatable.

The tissues of the vulva, vagina, cervix, or womb lining have thinned and become fragile, leaving them more prone to bleeding. This is the most prevalent cause of postmenopausal bleeding. There are more reasons as well, such as cervix or womb lining polyps. These are tiny growths, most of which are not malignant.

Perimenopause is when menopause-related period alterations first appear. Perimenopause normally begins eight to 10 years (though it might be shorter) before menopause, in your mid-to-late 40s (but it can start earlier or later for certain people).

Many women will use hormones to control their menstrual cycles, either as contraceptives or to treat endometriosis or heavy periods. Therefore, you cannot use altering bleeding patterns to determine whether you are in perimenopause or have gone through menopause if you are on hormones.

All women who are now experiencing periods eventually experience menopause, during which their periods cease. In the UK, menopause typically occurs at age 51, and by the time a woman reaches the age of 55, most women have ceased menstruating on their own.

How are menstrual changes handled?

A doctor should be consulted if:
You have heavier bleeding, your periods are lasting longer, you are bleeding in between periods, you have menopausal vaginal bleeding after sex, or you stop bleeding for a year or more before starting again.

A complete blood count and an assessment of your iron levels may also be necessary.

During perimenopause, irregular and severe bleeding can last for years. You might want to think about getting therapy to reduce or stop your menstruation. Options that can assist with this include both hormonal and non-hormonal ones:

Non-hormonal alternativesTranexamic acid: This pill is only to be used while bleeding. Mefenamic acid is a pill that is comparable to ibuprofen and aspirin. It is useful for period discomfort and can be successful in 'turning down the tap' and making periods lighter. Take this before and throughout bleeding.

GPs or our menopausal clinic can prescribe one of these choices.

Hormonal optionsThe progesterone-only pill - Although some women have more frequent bleeding, this option might be useful for those who experience severe menstrual bleeding. Since it's only a tablet, it's simple to start and stop. The combination pill is still a viable choice for certain women under the age of 50, and sequential HRT can be useful in controlling bleeding. However, it is not approved for use as part of HRT. It interferes with your hormones, resulting in a monthly bleed. You may.

MOODSWINGS

Estrogen levels fall during the menopausal transition, resulting in significant changes all over the body. Menopausal mood fluctuations are directly linked to several of these changes.

For instance, a decrease in estrogen may have an impact on how the body regulates the neurotransmitters serotonin and norepinephrine, which have been linked to depression. However, the evidence supporting this association is conflicting.

Lower estrogen levels are associated with irritation, exhaustion, stress, forgetfulness, anxiety, and trouble focusing.

There may be more than one direct cause-and-effect link between sadness, rage, and anxiety and the influence of these shifting hormone levels. Changes in hormone levels might make these symptoms worse.

Additionally, perimenopausal women have increased amounts of the brain protein monoamine oxidase A (MAO-A), according to a study. The depressed symptoms of this protein have been linked.

Reactions can compound, as is the case with night sweats. When someone is sleeping, they experience these hot flashes. A person may wake up in the middle of the night due to severe night sweats. Multiple nights of interrupted sleep can lead to irritation, muddled thinking, and other symptoms of menopausal mood swings.

risk elements

A history of severe premenstrual syndrome (PMS) and previous experiences of depression or other serious mental health issues are two of the key risk factors for unpleasant menopausal mood swings.

People may also be more vulnerable to emotional issues during menopause if they experience any of the following:

connections with loved ones that need improvement
a lot of stress in their daily lives
a challenging home scenario

Menopause mood swings can have a variety of more common effects, including:

Depression: One common and severe emotional side effect of menopause is depression. As they move through menopause, up to 1 in 5 Trusted sources experience it.

Anxiety: During menopause, many individuals suffer tension, anxiousness, concern, and panic attacks. While some people may notice an increase in their anxiety, others could experience it for the first time.

poor self-esteem: During and after menopause, people may suffer poor self-esteem and bad mood. Some people may experience higher levels of emotion or stronger reactions to circumstances.

Irritability: During the early menopausal transition, many persons notice an increase in their level of irritability.

Complications

Some people may choose to "self-medicate" with alcohol or other substances to deal with the shifting landscape of their life and the mood swings associated with menopause.

Unfortunately, these decisions make it more challenging for them to confront and address their worries. Additionally, it could raise the issue of substance abuse for them to confront.

INSOMNIA

Unwanted yet frequently occurring, insomnia is a side effect of menopause. Here, we examine the problem of menopausal sleeplessness and provide some potential remedies.
Every woman will experience menopause as a natural part of aging, but most of us would like to avoid some of the symptoms.

One of them is insomnia, which is the persistent inability to fall or stay asleep.

You have insomnia if you frequently have problems falling asleep. You can have trouble going to sleep, keeping asleep, or waking up still feeling weary.

Although many individuals experience insomnia, getting it as you age is more common. Additionally, it's typical for sleep issues to worsen if you're going through menopause or the perimenopause period.

What results in sleeplessness during menopause?
Your estrogen levels alter and steadily decline during perimenopause and menopause.

Not only may these hormonal shifts create sleep problems, but they can also induce additional symptoms including mood swings, night sweats, and hot flashes.

During perimenopause, hot flashes and nocturnal sweats in particular are a frequent cause of sleeplessness.

Additionally, there are other potential causes of your sleeplessness at this period of your life that are unrelated to hormone changes. These include both physical ailments like long-term (chronic) pain, obstructive sleep apnea, restless legs syndrome, anxiety, or depression, as well as psychological ones like work stress, money concerns, or relationship challenges.

How long does sleeplessness with menopause last?
If your sleeplessness is caused by menopause's hormonal changes, it will usually gradually go away once your hormones have normalized, but this process might take a while. If you don't take action to control it, it may persist for months or even years if it is brought on by other issues.

What causes my menopausal night sweats?

Hot flushes known as night sweats frequently cause you to wake up with sweat-covered sheets and nightclothes. While it is known that other factors, such as illness and lifestyle choices, can also cause them, during the menopausal years, estrogen imbalances are frequently to blame[2]. Decreasing levels of estrogen can have an impact on your body's internal thermostat, leading it to believe that you are too warm. Your body then tries to expel the extra heat by widening the blood vessels close to the head, neck, and chest, which can result in hot flashes at any moment. Even though night sweats may not alter how much sleep you get overall, they might disturb your sleep cycle by forcing you to wake up during the night, which can leave you feeling exhausted and anxious.

Making a few modest adjustments to your nightly routine and surroundings might make a big difference. Our cooling nightgowns and other lightweight, moisture-wicking clothes may keep your skin feeling cool and dry. A fan next to your bed, a big glass of cold water, and breathable linens designed to keep you warm and comfortable all night are further suggestions. Avoiding hot flash triggers like alcohol, caffeine, and spicy food can also be quite effective.

Why do I feel itchy all night?

One fairly unanticipated and less-discussed side-effect of menopause is itchy skin (pruritus). The capacity of our skin to renew and keep its natural oils and moisture is impacted by declining estrogen levels throughout menopause, leading to thinner, drier skin that can feel irritated and itchy, even at sleep. Many menopausal women may therefore suffer skin sensitivity all over their bodies, including their arms, legs, chest, back, and even vagina.

Even while these aging-related changes to our skin are unavoidable, there are various ways to calm your skin and get rid of the itching that's keeping you up at night, including dietary modifications, natural home remedies, and medical procedures. Collagen peptides, vitamins C, D, E, and K, and collagen all play crucial roles in the health of your skin. These nutrients may be found in over-the-counter supplements, however, you can also acquire them through food. Some clothing items, like our own HydraDerma line, are specially made to provide your skin with an additional layer of protection. This helps to increase moisture retention and lessen irritation during this normally difficult period.

Sleeping well through the menopausal transition
To enhance your sleep during and after the menopause transition:

Maintain a consistent sleep routine. Set a consistent wake-up and sleep time each day. If you can, try to avoid taking naps in the late afternoon or evening. It might cause you to lose sleep.
Set up a nighttime schedule. Some individuals unwind by reading a book, taking a warm bath, or listening to calming music.
Try to avoid using your computer, phone, or television in your bedroom. You can have trouble falling asleep due to the brightness of these devices.
Maintain a calm environment and a reasonable room temperature in your bedroom.

Exercise regularly throughout the day, but not right before bed.

Avoid eating a lot right before bed.

Avoid consuming caffeine late in the day (it may be found in a lot of coffee, tea, and chocolate).

Don't forget that drinking won't make you sleepy. It's challenging to stay asleep even in little doses.

WEIGHT GAIN

Menopause is typically not thought to be the primary cause of weight increase between the ages of 45 and 55, while additional study is required. But the drop in estrogen levels that comes with menopause can help in a few different ways.

The first effect of estrogen on the body is to increase muscle mass, which has an impact on metabolism, or how your body consumes energy. You're more likely to experience a slowed metabolism during perimenopause and when you reach menopause since less estrogen equals less muscle mass. You don't need as many calories to maintain the same weight if your metabolism is slower.

Combining this with a decline in muscle mass can result in higher levels of body fat and a heavier appearance, even without a weight change. Decreased estrogen can also cause your body to start storing more fat in your abdomen than in other areas of your body; this is known as the "menopause belly."

There are additional elements that support menopausal weight gain.
Weight gain during and after menopause is more frequently linked to aging and lifestyle factors. Aging naturally results in declines in muscle mass and metabolism, similar to changes in hormones. Therefore, it becomes particularly simple to consume more calories than your body requires and to store those additional calories as fat.

However, lifestyle elements like what you eat, how much you consume, and how much exercise you receive might have the most impact on your weight.

Chapter 3 Menopause treatments

Hormone Replacement Therapy (HRT)

a. Estrogen Therapy: Women who have had a hysterectomy (the surgical removal of the uterus) can benefit from estrogen-only therapy. Hot flashes, nocturnal sweats, vaginal dryness, and urinary symptoms can all be successfully treated with it.

b. Estrogen-Progestin Therapy: Women who still have an intact uterus might consider this combo therapy. To shield the uterine lining from the possible dangers of estrogen treatment alone, progestin is added.

Non-Hormonal Medications

a.   Serotonin-Norepinephrine   Reuptake Inhibitors (SNRIs) and Selective Serotonin Reuptake Inhibitors (SSRIs): These drugs, which   are   frequently   used   as antidepressants, have been useful in easing hot flashes and other depressive symptoms. Gabapentin, b. Gabapentin, which was first discovered to treat neuropathic pain and seizure disorders, is now shown to lessen both the frequency and intensity of hot flashes.

Vaginal Estrogen Therapy

a. Creams: To treat symptoms including vaginal dryness, itching, and discomfort during sex, vaginal estrogen creams are administered directly to the vaginal walls.

b. pills: To enhance vaginal health, vaginal estrogen pills are put into the vagina and gradually release estrogen.

c. Vaginal estrogen rings are put into the vagina and deliver estrogen continuously for a certain amount of time, usually three months.

Changes in Lifestyle

Regular exercise can improve mood, lessen hot flashes, encourage better sleep, and maintain general health, all of which can assist manage menopausal symptoms.

b. Healthful Diet: During menopause, a well-balanced diet full of fruits, vegetables, whole grains, lean proteins, and healthy fats can promote general well-being.

c. Stress management: Deep breathing, mindfulness, meditation, yoga, and other practices can help lower stress and enhance emotional well-being.

d. Avoiding Triggers: Reducing the frequency and intensity of hot flashes can be achieved by identifying and avoiding hot flash triggers such as spicy foods, caffeine, alcohol, and tight clothes.

Alternative Medicine

a. Acupuncture: In this kind of traditional Chinese treatment, tiny needles are inserted into the body at particular locations to treat menopausal symptoms.

b. Herbal Treatments: Some herbal remedies, such as dong quai, black cohosh, and soy products, have been used to treat menopausal symptoms. However, given their efficacy and safety might differ, it's crucial to speak with a healthcare provider before utilizing any herbal therapies.

c. Mind-Body Techniques: Activities like guided imagery, meditation, and relaxation techniques can all assist to lower stress levels, encourage relaxation, and enhance general well-being.

Each woman's experience with menopause is unique, and the therapy chosen should be based on her specific requirements, preferences, and health considerations. There are several ways to properly treat menopausal symptoms, including hormone replacement therapy, non-hormonal medicines, vaginal estrogen treatment, lifestyle changes, and complementary therapies. It is crucial to speak with a healthcare expert to go through the advantages, disadvantages, and applicability of various therapies based on your unique situation.

Natural Solutions

Women who choose a more holistic approach or who are unable to undergo hormone replacement treatment might manage menopausal symptoms with natural medicines. Although these treatments might not be effective for everyone, they are usually secure and worth taking into account. Here are a few all-natural treatments for menopause:

1. Phytoestrogens are plant chemicals that have actions similar to those of estrogen in the body. Soybeans, tofu, tempeh, flaxseeds, sesame seeds, and legumes are foods high in phytoestrogens. Your diet may benefit from including these items to aid with hot flashes, vaginal dryness, and mood swings.

2. Black cohosh: This herb is frequently used to treat hot flashes, mood swings, and insomnia brought on by menopause. Although its mode of action is unclear, it is thought to have estrogen-like actions. Before consuming black cohosh, it's crucial to speak with a doctor, especially if you have a history of liver issues.

3. Dong quai: Also referred to as female ginseng, dong quai is a herb that has been used in traditional Chinese medicine to regulate hormone levels and treat

menopausal symptoms. It is frequently advised for mood swings, vaginal dryness, and hot flashes. It should be taken cautiously, especially if you have a bleeding disease or are using blood-thinning drugs, as it, like black cohosh, may have an impact on blood coagulation.

4. Evening Primrose Oil: Made from the evening primrose plant, this oil includes the omega-6 fatty acid gamma-linolenic acid (GLA). Hot flashes, mood swings, and breast soreness may all be reduced by it. However, there is little scientific proof of its efficacy, and individual outcomes may differ.

5. Vitamin E: According to some research, vitamin E may help menopausal women have fewer and milder hot flashes. You may either buy it as a supplement or get it from foods like almonds, sunflower seeds, spinach, and avocados. Find out from your healthcare professional what dose is right for you.

6. Regular Physical Activity: Menopausal symptoms, such as hot flashes, mood fluctuations, weight gain, and sleep difficulties, can be managed with regular physical activity. On most days of the week, try to get in at least 30 minutes of moderate-intensity activity, such as brisk walking, swimming, or cycling.

7. Stress Reduction Strategies: Stress might make symptoms of menopause worse. Deep breathing, meditation, yoga, and other stress-reduction practices can aid in promoting relaxation, enhancing sleep, and lowering anxiety.

It's crucial to remember that natural therapies come in different safety and efficacy levels, and they may not work for everyone. Before beginning any new natural therapies, it is advised to speak with a healthcare provider or licensed naturopathic doctor, especially if you have any underlying medical concerns or are using other drugs.

Slow the aging process

Even though menopause affects half of the world's population, it is rarely talked about how it affects health and lifespan. What is ovarian aging, and how may it be postponed?

The end of a woman's reproductive years is indicated by the onset of menopause in middle age. Menopause can be freeing, but it can also cause health problems. Ovarian aging leads to menopause, which is also linked to several age-related disorders. Menopause is rarely acknowledged although impacting 50% of the world's population. How can we prevent menopause, what causes it, and how does it impact our health and longevity?

Menopause is mostly brought on by ovarian age. The eggs needed for reproduction develop in the ovaries. Ovaries age like all other parts of our body. It's interesting to note that the ovaries age twice as quickly as other bodily tissues, making them the body's first to show signs of aging. As they may also accelerate the aging of other bodily organs, they are regarded as the pacemaker of female aging.

The hormone estrogen is mostly produced by the ovaries. Estrogen levels decrease with aging. The amount and quality of the eggs produced by the ovaries also gradually deteriorate with time, finally resulting in infertility and menopause at an average age of 45 to 55.

What impact does menopause have on longevity and health?

For female fertility and health, it is crucial to stop or postpone ovarian aging. Many women are opting to put off having children as a result of their increased participation in the job, education, and financial independence during the previous century. Some people who ultimately decide to have children have trouble getting pregnant naturally beyond the age of 35. In addition to easing the societal and reproductive pressure to have children before 35, delaying ovarian aging would make it simpler for women to opt to have children later in life.

Health and lifespan may suffer greatly as a result of menopause. Menopause has a long-term effect on health and longevity in addition to the frequent symptoms that may be managed with hormone replacement therapy (HRT). Women's life expectancy has increased dramatically by 30 years, yet menopause has only been postponed by a meager 4 years. This implies that many women suffer from poor health for years on end. This is a problem of inequality since, even though women live longer than men do internationally, they also have poorer health 34% of the time, as opposed to 26% for men.

Increased risk for several age-related illnesses, including cardiovascular disease, frailty, and Alzheimer's, which can shorten lifespan, occurs with menopause. The decrease in estrogen, which controls the metabolic system, is to blame for this.

Hormones maintain a fine line between being beneficial to health and being harmful. Menopause-related low estrogen levels have been associated to cardiovascular illness, but the contraceptive pill's excessive estrogen levels have been connected to an increased risk of cancer, blood clots, and stroke. Estrogen has a variety of roles in the body that scientists are still learning about.

prevention of ovarian aging

Fortunately, there are a variety of treatments available for menopause's transient symptoms. HRT is a popular alternative that uses synthetic hormones to replace low levels of natural ones. It is often administered as a tablet, gel, patch, or implant. Hot flashes, mental dullness, and mood swings can all be helped by this. Long-term conditions linked to menopause, such as osteoporosis and heart disease, may be prevented by it as well. However, there is some evidence that certain HRTs may modestly raise the risk of cancer, blood clots, and stroke, just like the contraceptive pill does.

In addition to medication, lifestyle changes that might improve health as you age are frequently prescribed by doctors for menopausal symptoms:

To reduce the risk of osteoporosis, eat a balanced diet that is high in calcium-rich foods such as milk, yogurt, and kale.Rest and have a regular sleep schedule regular exercise will help you gain strength and muscle.

They also advise against smoking and consuming too much alcohol.

The goal of many businesses in the longevity sector is to combat ovarian aging, which is the primary cause of menopause and infertility. The answer could be in longevity pills. The nine signs of aging that affect the ovaries are the focus of several potential therapies. As an illustration, oxidative stress brought on by free radicals is regarded to be the primary cause of ovarian aging. It has been proposed to lessen this kind of stress by employing antioxidants, which are found in longevity supplements like curcumin, coenzyme Q10, and the hormone melatonin. NAD+ precursors like NR and NMN may be an alternative because it has been demonstrated that NAD+ can restore female fertility as people age.

Supplements that resemble fasting and calorie restriction through fasting have also been recommended, although there is conflicting information about whether these strategies slow down the aging of the ovaries. Platelet-rich plasma (PRP) blood transfers, stem cell treatments, and gene therapies are some further experimental concepts. These are still in their early phases, though. Until then, maintaining a healthy lifestyle, maybe assisted by supplements, appears to be essential for coping with ovarian aging and menopause.

Chapter 4 menopause-related memory loss (Brain fog)

The phrase "brain fog" is used to describe several symptoms that impair your capacity to think clearly, such as memory loss or difficulty concentrating. Although forgetfulness and memory lapses are frequently mistaken for signs of aging, they can also occur during menopause.

According to one research, memory deficits peak during perimenopause, which can persist for anywhere between 4 and 12 years, and affect about 60% of middle-aged women.

Brain fog is a menopausal symptom, just like hot flashes, mood swings, and sleeplessness, and it should be addressed as such rather than minimized or discounted. It's vital to keep in mind that you're not the only one going through the menopausal brain fog and that there is support accessible. Here, we look at a few strategies for controlling your symptoms.

Menopausal brain fog: What is it?

The simplest way to describe menopausal brain fog is as a "cotton wool" feeling. You might find it difficult to remember and retain knowledge or to focus on easy chores. Common concerns include forgetting what you were doing when you entered a room or having trouble recalling your neighbor's name.

After suffering from brain fog, some women may worry about getting dementia or Alzheimer's. Evidence, however, shows that memory and learning skills increase after menopause: in 2009, researchers examined more than 2,000 women over four years and discovered that cognitive problems improved after menopause.

When does menopause-related mental fog begin?

As a result of the fact that every woman's body will respond differently to the many ways her hormones fluctuate throughout perimenopause, there is no certain method to predict when or whether you may have menopausal brain fog. The first year following the last menstrual cycle (postmenopause), according to studies, is when some decline in cognitive performance (attention/working memory, verbal learning, verbal memory, and fine motor skill) are most noticeable.

What is the root cause of menopausal fog?

Since the hormones estrogen, progesterone, follicle-stimulating hormone (FSH), and luteinizing hormone (LH) all affect cognition, researchers believe that the perimenopausal hormone fluctuations that cause brain fog are to blame.

Although additional menopausal symptoms including hot flashes, night sweats, trouble sleeping, anxiety, and depression may also affect memory, they don't seem to be the main factor in brain fog. Instead, research appears that menopausal women are more prone to experience cognitive difficulties as a result of hormonal changes, particularly those brought on by estrogen.

How to deal with menopausal fog

Given that the human brain is mostly made up of water (75%), even very slight dehydration can impair cognitive abilities and cause problems with memory and focus.

Make a deliberate effort to increase your daily water intake. When you first get up in the morning, drink two glasses of water. You may also set an alarm to remind you to get up from your desk and drink a glass of water every hour. To add taste and make your drink more flavorful and refreshing, you may add lemon, mint, or cucumber.

Add extra beneficial fats.

A healthy diet should always be maintained for cognitive function. Due to the presence of omega-3 fatty acids and unsaturated fats in the Mediterranean diet, these nutrients have been extensively praised for their ability to protect the brain. According to empirical evidence, consuming a mostly Mediterranean diet is associated with a decreased risk of cognitive impairment and a slower pace of cognitive aging.

Increase your intake of vegetables, fruits, legumes, nuts, beans, grains, cereals, oily fish (such as mackerel, salmon, herring, and anchovies), and unsaturated fats (such as olive oil, avocado, and almonds) to boost your cognitive health.

Engage in routine workout

Menopause symptoms, especially those related to cognition, can be effectively managed by engaging in regular exercise. According to one study, high-intensity exercise may boost information processing speed, whereas moderate-intensity exercise may promote cognitive flexibility and working memory.

At least five days a week, try to get in 30 minutes of moderately intense cardiovascular activity. Try to pick an activity you love, such as dance, swimming, power walking, running, or cycling.

Strength training is something else you may think about including in your fitness routine. Aim for two weightlifting or calisthenics exercises each week, including squats, lunges, and pushups.

Get enough sleep.

For optimal cognitive performance, getting adequate good sleep is also crucial. Rapid eye movement (REM) sleep, which occurs in the later phases of your sleep cycle, is when your brain consolidates thoughts, retains memories, and absorbs information from the previous day.

However, many menopausal women also have insomnia as a result of erratic hormone levels, which is still additional justification for prioritizing your sleep hygiene.

Give yourself enough time to relax before bed because stress and worry can make sleeping problems worse. You may think about doing yoga, deep breathing exercises, meditation, or taking a hot bath.

Make sure that your bedroom is between 16 and 18 degrees, dress comfortably, and stay away from heavy duvets or blankets to prevent night sweats from interfering with your sleep.

Finally, try to avoid consuming heavy meals, coffee, nicotine, or alcohol just before bed because these can interfere with your ability to fall asleep and the quality of your sleep.

Including soy isoflavones

Soy and other phytoestrogens have shown promise in enhancing general health and cognitive performance after menopause. If you don't like soy-based foods, you might want to supplement your diet with soya isoflavones.

Consider ginkgo biloba.

Ginkgo biloba is a well-liked herbal remedy for treating menopausal symptoms. There is some evidence to support the idea that ginkgo biloba may support short-term memory and sustain normal cognitive function.

We recognize that memory loss and brain fog can be frightening but be reassured that menopausal symptoms frequently get better with time, particularly if you work to promote your general cognitive health.

However, it's crucial to consult your doctor if your symptoms are impairing your quality of life or don't go away.

Chapter 5 Healthy forever: menopause and Beyond

- Exercise

- Adults should engage in at least 150 minutes of moderate-intensity activity or 75 minutes of vigorous-intensity exercise per week, according to the NHS guidelines. This especially applies to women who are going through menopause. You have the option of doing all of your weekly workouts at once, in short sessions, or a combination of both.

- What is mild, medium, and strong intensity?

- Your heart rate should increase with moderately intense activity. You can converse but not sing as your breathing gets deeper. Examples include cycling, water aerobics, fast walking, and even pulling a lawnmower.

- When you engage in vigorous activity, your breathing alters and you can only speak briefly in between breaths. There are several alternatives, including running, swimming, hockey, football, netball, rapid cycling, aerobics, and swimming.

- benefits of exercise for health

- Increasing bone mass

- During menopause, when estrogen levels fall, we begin to absorb bone minerals more quickly than we can create them. As a result, there is a decrease in bone density, which may lead to osteoporosis. 536,000 persons in the UK, or one in three menopausal women, may get an osteoporotic fracture each year.

- The good news is that low-impact, weight-bearing exercise can raise bone density. It's never too late to start because research indicates that a progressive resistance training program performed for at least four to six months can favorably affect bone density. Weight-bearing exercises include walking, stair climbing, dancing, leaping, and jogging. Lifting weights, using resistance bands, or even utilizing your body weight, such as when performing press-ups, are all examples of muscle-strengthening activities. Strength exercises should be done two to three times a week, according to the Royal Osteoporosis Society. Sitting or rising from your chair eight to twelve times without moving your arms might be considered an easy activity.

- Circulatory System
- This is your heart, blood arteries, and the blood that flows through them, to put it simply. Estrogen contributes to the maintenance of a healthy system by keeping the blood vessels flexible and by assisting in cholesterol management. Women are more susceptible to high blood pressure, plaque buildup, coronary heart disease, high blood pressure, heart attacks, and stroke when estrogen levels decline.

- Your cardiovascular system will benefit if you exercise at the suggested level by the NHS each week. Under the heading "What exactly is moderate and vigorous intensity?" a few examples were provided.

- Bringing Down Cortisol Levels

- Your stress hormone, cortisol, can disrupt the harmony of your hormones, worsen menopausal symptoms, and lead to abdominal fat deposition along with low estrogen levels. These may have been distributed more uniformly before the menopause.

- Exercise releases endorphins, or "feel good" chemicals, which help you feel better, burn calories, and reduce stress by lowering the amount of the stress hormone cortisol. Stress-reduction methods including breathing exercises, yoga, and meditation are highly effective (see the section below on mental health).

- In conclusion, cardiovascular issues may be avoided by engaging in activity that increases your heart rate and strengthens your cardiovascular system. Training with weights or resistance bands increases muscle and bone strength, lowering the chance of fracture and boosting metabolism, both of which will help with the spread of midlife fat deposits.

- Finding workouts you love performing is crucial since you are more likely to keep up with them. You may begin exercising at any level and progressively increase your intensity over time.

- Nutrition
- Menopausal symptoms might be less severe with a good diet. Additionally, it will aid in preventing long-term health issues brought on by the absence of estrogens, such as heart disease, strokes, and a loss of bone density.
- To enhance your diet, you might want to give any of the following a try:
- For strong bones, eat a lot of foods high in calcium and vitamin D. You should be able to receive the 700 mg of calcium per day suggested for the

country from your diet. Dairy products (low-fat), salmon and sardines in cans, green leafy vegetables, fortified bread, and morning cereals are all good sources.

- Vitamin D is encouraged to be produced by sunlight. This aids in the body's absorption of calcium, which is necessary for maintaining healthy bone density. From October to March in England, Wales, and Ireland, and all year in Scotland, a daily vitamin D pill of 10 micrograms is advised.

- Think about serving size. We require fewer calories as we age because our metabolic rate decreases. It has been demonstrated that being overweight worsens hot flashes and raises the risk of diabetes, heart disease, and vitamin D insufficiency. A smaller plate could be used to assist you manage your portions.

- Consume five servings or more of fruit and vegetables each day.

- Cut back on prepared meals and highly processed foods.

- Reduce refined carbs, especially sugary meals, which can cause your blood sugar to spike suddenly and then drop suddenly, leaving you feeling exhausted and hungry.

- Limit your salt consumption. A daily salt consumption of no more than 6 grams is advised.

- You might want to give foods containing phyto-estrogens (such as isoflavones or lignans) a try. They have a structure that is comparable to estrogen and may be useful for treating symptoms including hot flashes and vaginal dryness. Soybeans, green beans, lentils, chickpeas, textured vegetable protein, tofu, and soy beverages all contain isoflavones. Cereals, linseeds, fruit, and vegetables all contain lignans.

- Reduce your intake of alcohol and caffeine since these substances may aid to lessen night sweats and hot flashes. Additionally, possible mood-altering factors include caffeine, alcohol, spicy foods, and smoking. Overindulgence in alcohol increases the risk of fracture and osteoporosis. It is advised that women limit their weekly intake of alcohol to 14 units, with occasional days without it.

- Stop smoking. Smokers experience menopause sooner than non-smokers, experience more painful flushes, and frequently do not respond as well to HRT in tablet form. Smoking is damaging to your bones and prevents the development of bone density.
- The state of my mind

- The mental health of a woman may suffer throughout menopause. Some women describe feeling tense, irritable, moody, lethargic, or low in energy. These symptoms may have a direct or indirect impact on other aspects of your life, including sleep and interpersonal interactions. By adhering to the recommendations for exercise, nutrition, and sleep hygiene, try to stay on top of symptoms.

Cognitive Behavioural Therapy

- A quick, non-medical technique called cognitive behavior therapy (CBT) may be beneficial for a variety of mental health issues. CBT offers fresh coping mechanisms, and practical solutions, and aids in problem-solving for individuals. Managing stress and anxiety can assist with menopausal physical symptoms. Menopause does not create worry or tension, but you should think about what else could be going on in your life that might. Adolescent children, an elderly and unwell parent, or a shift in your social or professional life might be the cause of this.

- Mindfulness

- Another psychological tool for managing mental health is mindfulness.

- As a therapeutic method, mindfulness is a mental state attained by keeping one's attention on the present while calmly noticing and accepting one's feelings, thoughts, and physical sensations.

- According to some research, practicing mindfulness might help you feel less stressed and hence have fewer hot flashes. For additional details, please refer to the resources.

- Sleep

- Try to establish a schedule where you go to bed at the same time every night. Your body and mind will feel drowsy as a result at the appropriate moment. Make sure to provide the time required to get ready for your routine. To make up for this, you might have to go to bed sooner.

- Working or watching TV shouldn't be done in the bedroom. Remove all electronics to eliminate the temptation to check emails, including phones and PCs.

- Consider the environment. Reduce light, particularly "blue light" from phones and other devices, noise, and temperature to a comfortable level. A little colder environment might be beneficial.

- Try to leave at least a couple of hours between meals since eating too close to bedtime prevents your body from digesting a meal completely.

- Alcohol and caffeine can occasionally have a detrimental impact on how well you sleep. Keep an eye on what you're drinking and when.

- To guarantee that your body feels weary at night, make sure you exercise enough throughout the day. Don't "cat-nap" during the day or at night, if possible.

- If your mind is racing at night, try drafting a list of your concerns and promise yourself that you will take care of them in the morning. Write down your worries if they cause you to wake up in the middle of the night with anxiety so you can reflect on them the following day. So, keep a piece of paper and a pen beside your bed.

- Explore apps that can help you sleep such as 'Sleepio.'
- Sexual Behavior

- The vagina may alter as a result of menopause. Irritation, itching, and dryness in and around the vagina are common symptoms. This is quite uncomfortable for many women, and because of the pain it could cause, they frequently avoid having intimate relationships with their partners. 40% of menopausal women report having painful sex.

- Our ovaries quit producing estrogen, which causes this alteration in the tissues. Estrogen increases the suppleness and lubrication of the vaginal tissues. The tissues lose their suppleness and fatty tissue after depletion, becoming thin and friable. Menopausal women may encounter more urinary tract infections since the PH in the tissues also alters.

- Atrophic vaginitis, also known as vaginal atrophy, describes the changes in the vaginal lining that are frequently felt following menopause.

- In addition to estrogen, testosterone—which is responsible for libido, sexual desire, and the capacity for an orgasm—is also decreased during menopause.

- Our sexual life may be impacted in one way or another by the decline in both estrogen and testosterone throughout menopause. Some women can have urine urgency or stress incontinence in addition to these symptoms.

- Advice

- washing advice and hot flashes

- Keep scented lotions, fabric conditioners, and soaps to a minimum. Change your soap with an emollient wash.

-

- Avoid vaginal douching, which involves washing the interior of the vagina with water or another substance. It may change the PH balance in the tissues of the vagina, which may result in thrush or infections.

- You might want to consider your clothing choices if you frequently have hot flushes. Try wearing cotton, lighter-weight clothing, looser-fitting clothes, and maybe layers you can remove to help you cool down.
- Virility dryness
- Use a particular vaginal moisturizer to address this. Refrain from experimenting with lotions that you would normally use on other regions of your body. Vaginal moisturizers can be purchased without a prescription, online, or at retail stores.

- Make sure to use estrogen pessaries, cream, or the Estring (a soft ring worn within the vagina for three months that gently distributes a small dosage of estrogen straight to the vagina to alleviate dryness) to cure the vaginal atrophy. Your doctor may recommend them. Long-term usage is required for them.

- Additionally, a lubricant can enhance the comfort of sexual activity. Vaginal lubrication declines and the vaginal tissues dry down when natural estrogen levels are low. A lubricant used during sexual activity may help to counteract these alterations, which can reduce the pleasure of sexual penetration.

- Avoid unwelcome glycerin and parabens by using a water- or oil-based lubricant.

- KY Jelly, a lubricant, and moisturizer used for vaginal inspection, is NOT recommended. It is advisable to stay away from it as it includes chemicals that, if used frequently, might irritate the skin.

- Learning to relax your pelvic floor muscles might assist if you suffer discomfort during sex since your pelvic floor may be contracting excessively to 'defend' your vagina. The defensive guarding system may become active in response to vaginal discomfort or irritability. To learn how to relax the pelvic floor muscles, you might need to consult a physiotherapist who specializes in pelvic health.

- Maintain open lines of communication with your spouse so they are aware of how you are feeling and how it is affecting you.
- Talk to a trustworthy buddy about your problems as well; sharing your knowledge is beneficial.

- With your doctor, go through various hormone replacement therapy (HRT) alternatives.

- Avoid suffering alone.
- Exercises for the rectus muscles
- To support you, halt any urine leaks when you cough or sneeze, and help avoid prolapses, your pelvic floor muscles must be able to function effectively. You can have more sex and more orgasms if you have strong muscles. The Squeezy app is a

fantastic tool for strengthening these muscles.

- If you have symptoms of urinary incontinence or prolapse and they are not getting better, please contact your doctor for more assistance or self-refer to physiotherapy.